SOMATIC EXERCISES FOR WEIGHT LOSS

The Comprehensive Guide to Somatic Practices, Diet, and Well-being

BETH JAMES

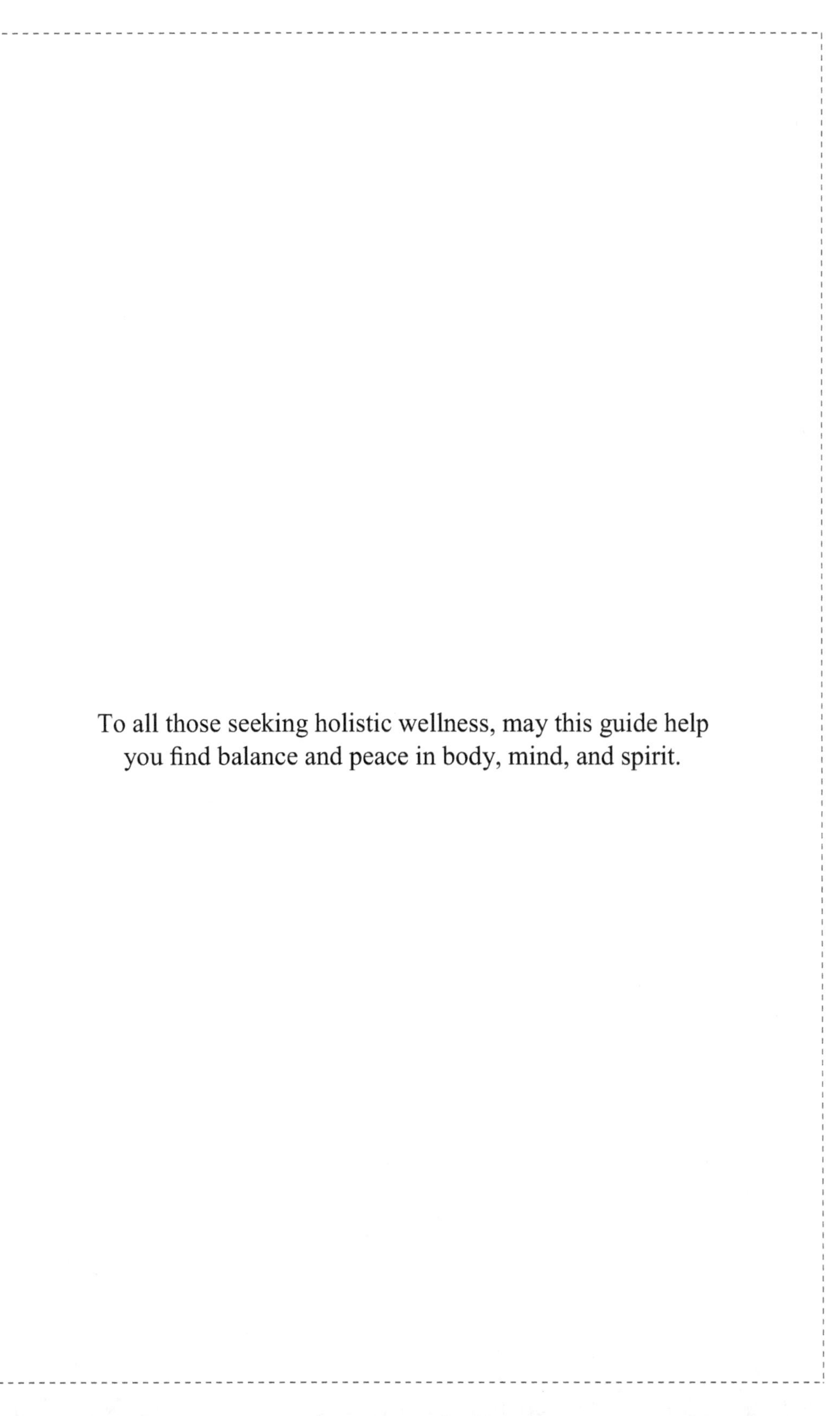

To all those seeking holistic wellness, may this guide help you find balance and peace in body, mind, and spirit.

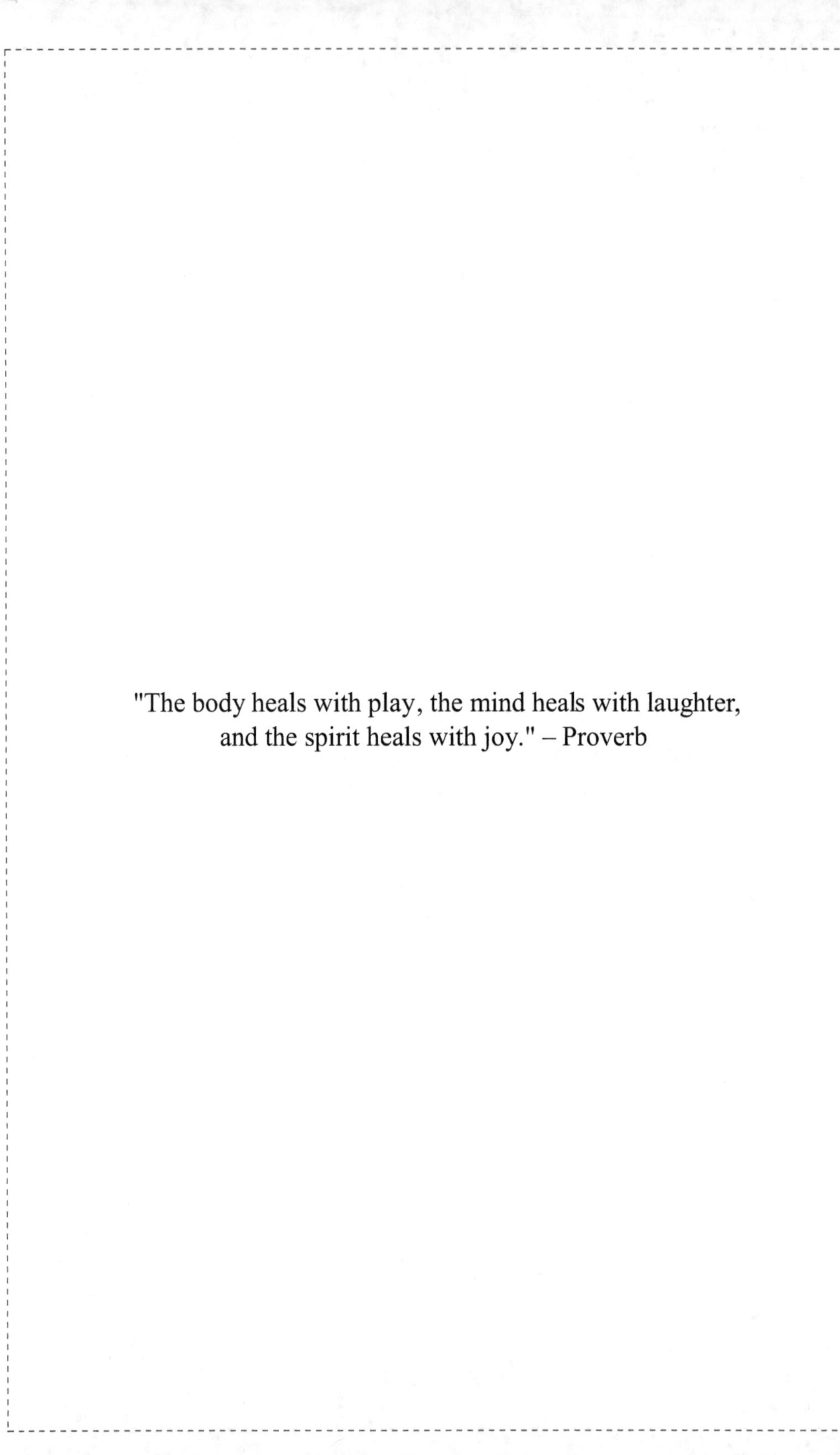

"The body heals with play, the mind heals with laughter,
and the spirit heals with joy." – Proverb

Table of Contents

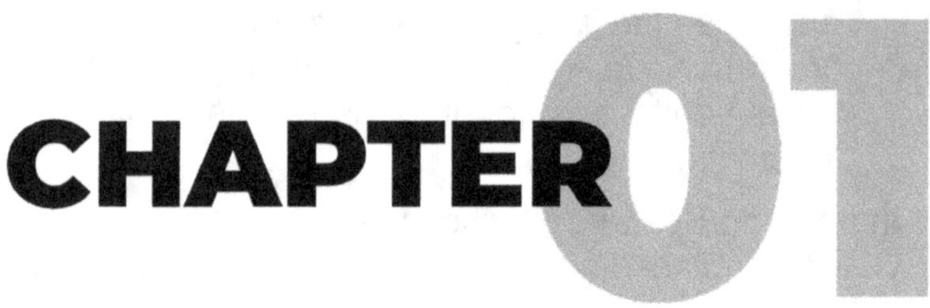

INTRODUCTION TO SOMATIC EXERCISES AND HOLISTIC WEIGHT LOSS

Get ready to start your path to a healthier and more balanced life. Let's explore somatic exercises and holistic weight loss together. We'll look at how these methods go beyond regular ones to boost emotional health and help manage stress.

What are Somatic Exercises?

Somatic exercises offer a fresh and life-changing way to get fit. They focus on how movement and sensation feel inside, not on outside results. Unlike usual exercises that track weight, reps, and speed, somatic exercises zero in on how your body feels as it moves. This focus on connecting mind and body helps you become more aware of your physical feelings. As a result, you can improve your coordination, balance, and overall health.

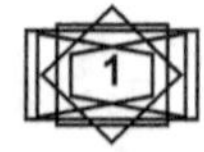

Origin and Evolution

The concept of somatic exercises has deep roots in various holistic practices that recognize the interconnectedness of the body and mind. The term "somatic" itself comes from the Greek word "soma," meaning "body," but in the context of these exercises, it encompasses the totality of one's physical and internal experiences. Influences from yoga, Tai Chi, the Feldenkrais Method, the Alexander Technique, and modern somatic therapies have converged to create a rich blend of practices that form the foundation of somatic exercises.

With its ancient tradition of combining physical postures, breath control, and meditation, yoga has significantly shaped the development of somatic exercises. Similarly, Tai Chi, with its slow, deliberate movements and focus on internal energy (qi), has contributed to the somatic understanding of mindful movement. The Feldenkrais Method and Alexander Technique, both developed in the 20th century, emphasize re-educating the body through movement to overcome pain and improve function, aligning perfectly with somatic principles.

Importance in Modern Health and Wellness

In today's fast-paced and often stressful world, somatic exercises offer a refreshing and necessary shift from the high-intensity, goal-oriented fitness routines that dominate the industry. These exercises are particularly beneficial for addressing modern health challenges such as chronic stress, anxiety, and sedentary lifestyles.

By fostering a deeper awareness of bodily sensations, somatic exercises help individuals recognize and release physical and emotional tension. This process can lead to improved posture, reduced pain, and a greater sense of ease and relaxation in everyday movements. Moreover, the mindful nature of somatic exercises encourages a more compassionate and patient relationship with one's body, which is crucial for sustainable weight loss and long-term health.

Mindful Movement and Breath Work

Central to somatic exercises are the practices of mindful movement and breath work. These elements are designed to cultivate a heightened state of awareness and presence, allowing individuals to connect deeply with their bodies and the present moment.

Mindful movement

Mindful movement means doing exercises while paying full attention to your body's signals and feedback. Instead of pushing through pain, you learn to move in ways that feel natural and good for you. This can be as simple as walking and paying attention to each step or doing gentle stretches that focus on smooth and easy motions.

Breath Work

Breathwork, or conscious breathing, is another vital part of somatic exercises. When you focus on your breath, you can influence your nervous system, lower stress, and boost your overall feeling of well-being. Methods like diaphragmatic breathing, where you take deep breaths into your belly, or

alternate nostril breathing, can help calm your mind and balance your body's energy.

Integrating Mindful Movement and Breath Work

The combination of mindful movement and breath work influences each other, enhancing the advantages of both practices. For example, matching your breathing to your movements, as you see in yoga or Tai Chi, can strengthen your body awareness and boost the impact of each exercise. This blend helps to create a well-rounded workout plan that supports not just physical health but also improves emotional and mental wellness. This mix nurtures your overall well-being, going beyond just physical fitness to enrich your mind and emotions.

Real-Life Application

Picture this: You start your day with some easy, mindful stretches. You stand with your feet hip-width apart and take a few deep breaths to center yourself. As you breathe in, you lift your arms above your head, feeling the stretch in your sides and back. When you breathe out, you lower your arms, noticing how your shoulders relax. This simple routine doesn't just wake up your body - it also sets a thoughtful mood for the day. It helps you to approach meals, work, and conversations with more calm and awareness.

By making these practices part of your everyday routine, you can change how you approach weight loss and wellness. You'll go beyond the strict rules of regular workout plans and build a more flexible, intuitive, and kind relationship with your body. This path of body awareness isn't just about shedding pounds; it helps you understand yourself better and lays the groundwork for long-term health and joy.

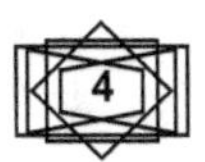

Understanding Weight Loss Beyond the Scale

Kicking off a weight loss plan can seem like it's all about the numbers, with the scale acting as a harsh critic of whether you're winning or losing. But real, lasting weight loss is about way more than what that machine tells you. In this part, we'll look at the big-picture approach to dropping pounds, showing how it covers physical health, feelings, and mental wellness.

Holistic Weight Loss: A Comprehensive Approach (Physical, Emotional, and Psychological Well-being)

Holistic weight loss takes a full view of health. It goes beyond just losing pounds; it aims to nourish your whole self. This method shows that your physical health connects to how you feel and think. When your mind and emotions are in good shape, your body tends to follow.

Holistic weight loss pushes you to tune in to your body's signals, meet its needs, and build a kind relationship with yourself. This means seeing that your weight is one part of your health and putting all your focus on it can often make you feel upset and let down.

A Gentle Sustainable Approach

Sustainability stands as a key principle in holistic weight loss. Traditional methods to lose weight often require significant changes that people struggle to keep up with over time, resulting in the feared yo-yo dieting effect. On the other hand, a holistic view supports small, steady changes that match your body's natural patterns and requirements.

This could mean picking nutrient-rich foods you like, discovering exercises that feel good to you, and learning stress-busting tricks that suit you. It's about building a way of life you can stick with and enjoy, not just a quick fix.

Holistic weight loss also recognizes that your body weight changes over time. Things like stress, sleep, and hormone shifts can all have an impact on your weight. Rather than seeing these changes as failures, holistic weight loss prompts you to view them as natural variations and to react with compassion and adaptability.

Measuring Success Beyond the Scale:

When you take on a holistic approach to weight loss, success no longer hinges on just one number. Instead, it's gauged by a set of health indicators and lifestyle enhancements. Here are a few signs of progress in holistic weight loss:

1. **Better Health** Signs: Watch for shifts in your overall health, like lower blood pressure, better cholesterol numbers, tighter blood sugar control, and higher fitness levels. These signs give a fuller picture of your health than just weight

2. **Steadier Emotions:** See how your mood and feelings get better as you do body-focused exercises and pick up healthier habits. Less stress, sounder sleep, and a stronger sense of well-being all show you're heading in the right direction.
3. **Better Day-to-Day Life:** Notice how your daily life gets better. Can you move around more? Do you have more zip to do things you enjoy? Is your connection with food becoming more positive and less rigid?
4. **Body Awareness and Mindfulness:** A vital part of holistic weight loss involves building a stronger bond with your body. When you do somatic exercises, you'll see your body awareness and mindfulness grow. This can lead you to eat and move in ways that are more intuitive and thoughtful.

Real-Life Application:

Think about Sarah, who started on a holistic path to lose weight. At first, she just wanted to shed pounds. But she soon learned that to change, she needed to think. She began to do somatic exercises. This helped her pay attention to how her body felt when she moved. Because of this, she started to pick exercises that made her feel good and were easy on her body instead of ones that hurt.

Sarah began to eat, paying attention to her feelings of hunger and fullness rather than counting calories. This change helped her build a better relationship with food. As time passed, she saw her mood improve, her energy increase, and her life quality get better overall. While the scale showed slow changes, she measured her success by how much better she felt in her body and mind.

The Science and Research That Supports Somatic Practices for Health

This section looks at the scientific basis of somatic exercises and shows their proven health and wellness benefits. By examining the research, we can gain a clearer understanding of how these practices can change your body and mind.

Somatic Practices and Their Benefits

Many studies show that somatic practices work well to boost overall health. These exercises focus on body awareness and thoughtful movement, and they have an impact on health in several ways:

Less Stress: Long-term stress can lead to many health issues, such as weight gain, heart disease, and mental health problems. Research proves that somatic practices can cut down stress levels a lot. Studies find that things like mindful movement and breathing exercises can lower cortisol—the stress hormone—in the body. This helps people feel more calm and balanced.

For example, a study in the *Journal of Alternative and Complementary Medicine* discovered that people who did somatic exercises felt less stressed and anxious. This drop in stress clears your mind and boosts your physical health, starting a good cycle that helps every part of your well-being.

Better Physical Function

Somatic exercises aim to improve how your body works by making you more aware of your movements and posture. This greater awareness can help you coordinate better, balance more easily, and become more flexible. It can also

lower your chance of getting hurt and make your body perform better overall.

A study in the *American Journal of Physical Medicine & Rehabilitation* showed that people who did somatic exercises got much better at moving and functioning. Older adults saw the most significant gains, which suggests somatic practices

could help people stay mobile and healthy as they age.

Clearer Thinking: To make smart choices about your health, you need a clear head. Somatic exercises can sharpen your mind and help you think more by getting you to focus on the present moment and be more aware.

Studies in *Frontiers in Psychology* revealed that people doing somatic exercises showed better attention, memory, and executive function. These brain boosts are connected to the practice's focus on careful attention and mindful awareness, which trains the brain to work more.

The Brain Science Behind Somatic Exercises

To get the power of somatic exercises, we need to understand how they affect our brains and nerves. These practices retrain the nervous system, boosting health and well-being in several key ways:

Retraining the Nervous System

Somatic exercises use the concept of neuroplasticity—the brain's ability to change itself by making new neural connections. When you practice mindful movement and body awareness, you can retrain your nervous system to adopt healthier patterns of movement and posture.

A study in *Neuroscience Letters* showed how somatic practices could change the brain. People who did regular mindful movement exercises had more connections in brain areas linked to sensory and motor function. These practices can boost the brain's ability to support physical and mental health.

Regulation of the Autonomic Nervous System

The autonomic nervous system (ANS) controls bodily functions we can't control on our own, like our heartbeat, digestion, and breathing rate. Somatic exercises can help balance the ANS, creating harmony between the sympathetic (fight or flight) and parasympathetic (rest and digest) parts.

A study in the *Journal of Psychophysiology* showed that somatic practices, breathing exercises, and mindful movement could boost parasympathetic activity. This shift towards a more balanced ANS can lower stress, help digestion, and support overall health.

Somatic Awareness and Weight Management

One of the most exciting things about somatic exercises is how they help with weight control. These practices help you become more aware of your body and eat more, which can lead to long-term weight loss and better overall health.

Better Eating Habits: When you're more aware of your body, you pay attention to when you're hungry or full. This makes it easier to eat and stop yourself from overeating. A study in the *Journal of Obesity* showed that people who practiced mindful eating, which is a big part of being aware of your body, lost a lot of weight and didn't binge eat as much.

Emotional Regulation: Many people trying to manage their weight face the challenge of emotional eating. Somatic exercises help control emotions by promoting mindfulness and body awareness. This makes it easier to spot and deal with emotional triggers that lead to overeating.

Research published in *the Appetite* journal showed that people who did somatic practices reported eating less due to emotions and feeling better about their body image. This control over emotions plays a crucial role in reaching and keeping a healthy weight.

Long-lasting Lifestyle Changes: Somatic exercises take a whole-person approach that supports lifestyle changes that stick. This method combines physical activity, mindfulness, and emotional health. It works better for keeping weight off in the long run compared to regular diet and exercise plans that often miss the link between mind and body.

A longitudinal study in *Health Psychology* showed that individuals who adopted a holistic approach, including somatic exercises, were more successful in maintaining their weight loss over time compared to those following conventional methods.

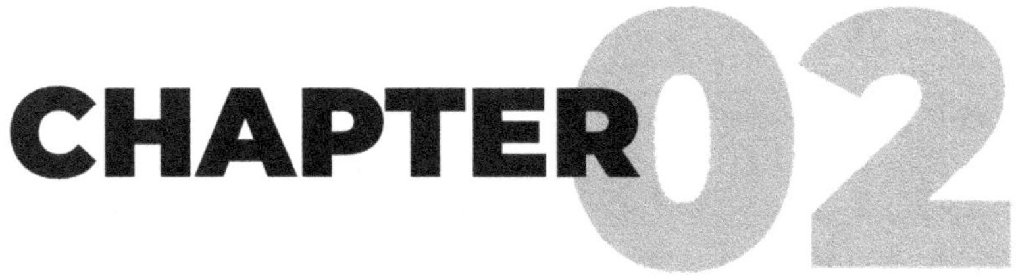

CHAPTER 02

THE CONNECTION BETWEEN MIND, BODY, AND WEIGHT MANAGEMENT

Welcome to a deeper dive into the fascinating interplay between your mind and body and how this connection plays a crucial role in weight management. This chapter is all about understanding the powerful relationship between mental, emotional, and physical health and how nurturing this relationship can lead to sustainable weight loss and overall well-being.

Exploring Body Awareness and Its Importance: Unlocking the Power of Body Awareness

Imagine being so in tune with your body that you can effortlessly distinguish between true hunger and a craving triggered by stress. This is the magic of body awareness, a

cornerstone of effective weight management and a vibrant, healthy life.

Recognizing Hunger and Satiety Cues

Body awareness starts with tuning into your body's natural signals. Many of us eat out of habit, stress, or boredom rather than genuine hunger. Developing body awareness helps you recognize true hunger and fullness cues, leading to healthier eating patterns. When you listen to your body, you learn to eat when you're genuinely hungry and stop when you're satisfied, which can naturally regulate your food intake and support weight loss.

For instance, imagine sitting down for a meal and taking a moment to breathe and center yourself. You pay attention to your stomach, noticing whether you're actually hungry or just eating because it's mealtime. This simple practice can revolutionize your eating habits, helping you make choices that nourish your body and align with your health goals.

Distinguishing Emotional vs. Physical Hunger

One of the most transformative aspects of body awareness is the ability to discern emotional hunger from physical hunger. Emotional hunger often comes on suddenly and is linked to specific cravings, usually for comfort foods. Physical hunger, on the other hand, builds gradually and can be satisfied with a variety of foods.

Enhanced somatic mindfulness—the practice of being fully present and aware of your body's sensations—can help you make this distinction. When you're mindful, you're more likely to pause and ask yourself if you're starving or if you're seeking food as a way to cope with emotions like stress, sadness, or boredom.

Consider this: You've had a stressful day at work, and you find yourself reaching for a sugary snack. By practicing somatic mindfulness, you pause and check in with your body. Are you physically hungry, or are you trying to soothe your emotions? This awareness can lead you to choose a different coping mechanism, such as taking a walk or practicing deep breathing, instead of turning to food.

Mitigating Chronic Pain and Improving Movement Efficiency

Body awareness isn't just about eating habits—it also plays a critical role in how you move and how you feel physically. Many people live with chronic pain or inefficient movement patterns that can make exercise challenging. By practicing body awareness, you can identify and address these issues, making physical activity more effective and enjoyable.

For example, somatic practices often include gentle movements that encourage you to explore how your body feels as it moves. These exercises can help you discover areas of tension or discomfort that you might not have noticed before. By addressing these issues, you can improve your movement efficiency, reduce pain, and enhance your overall physical function.

Imagine starting your day with a series of mindful stretches, paying close attention to how your body feels with each movement. You might notice tightness in your shoulders or stiffness in your lower back. By bringing awareness to these areas, you can begin to release tension and improve your range of motion, making your workouts more effective and reducing the risk of injury.

Real-Life Application:

Meet Alex, who struggled with emotional eating and chronic back pain. By incorporating body awareness practices into his daily routine, Alex learned to recognize when he was eating out of stress rather than hunger. He also discovered that his back pain was partly due to poor posture and inefficient movement patterns. Through somatic exercises and mindful eating, Alex not only lost weight but also experienced significant relief from his pain and an overall improvement in his quality of life.

How Emotional Balance Affects Weight

Welcome to an exploration of the profound connection between your emotional well-being and your physical health, particularly how it impacts weight management. In this section, we'll delve into the bidirectional relationship between emotional balance and body weight, highlighting how nurturing your emotional health can lead to positive changes in your physical health and vice versa.

The Impact of Emotional Distress on Weight

Life can be overwhelming, and it's natural to experience emotional distress from time to time. However, chronic emotional distress can significantly affect your weight management efforts. When you're feeling stressed, anxious, or depressed, you might turn to food for comfort—a behavior known as emotional eating. This can lead to overconsumption of unhealthy foods, which directly impacts your weight.

For instance, after a tough day, you might find yourself reaching for a tub of ice cream or a bag of chips, seeking solace in these comfort foods. While they might provide

temporary relief, they can also lead to unwanted weight gain and a cycle of guilt and further emotional distress.

The Role of Stable Emotional Health

Conversely, when your emotional health is stable, you're more likely to make consistent, healthful decisions about your diet and exercise. Emotional balance supports a clear mind, helping you to listen to your body's actual needs and make choices that align with your health goals.

Think about those days when you feel calm and centered. You're more likely to choose nutritious meals, exercise regularly, and practice self-care. These positive behaviors reinforce your emotional well-being, creating a beneficial cycle that supports both your mental and physical health.

Fostering Emotional Balance Through Somatic Practices

Here's the good news: practices that foster emotional balance, like somatic exercises, can help alleviate stress and reduce the likelihood of stress-induced eating. Somatic exercises emphasize the mind-body connection, promoting mindfulness and body awareness. These practices can be incredibly soothing, helping you to release tension and cultivate a sense of peace.

Stress Reduction: Somatic exercises, such as gentle stretching, deep breathing, and mindful movement, can significantly reduce stress levels. When you engage in these practices, you activate the body's relaxation response, lowering cortisol levels and promoting a state of calm. This can make a huge difference in how you handle daily stressors and can reduce the urge to turn to food for comfort.

Emotional Awareness: By enhancing your body awareness, somatic exercises help you become more attuned to your emotional states. You'll start to notice how different emotions manifest in your body—whether it's tightness in your chest, a knot in your stomach, or tension in your shoulders. This awareness allows you to address your emotions directly rather than masking them with food.

Mindful Eating: Practicing somatic mindfulness can also improve your eating habits. When you eat mindfully, you pay full attention to the experience of eating, noticing the flavors, textures, and sensations. This practice helps you recognize true hunger and fullness cues, making it easier to stop eating when you're satisfied rather than eating to soothe emotions.

Real-Life Application:

Meet Lisa, who struggled with emotional eating for years. By incorporating somatic exercises into her routine, she learned to manage her stress more effectively and became more aware of her emotional triggers. Instead of reaching for snacks when she felt anxious, Lisa started practicing deep breathing and gentle stretches. Over time, she noticed a significant improvement in her emotional health and a more balanced approach to eating.

Case Studies: Success Stories of Holistic Weight Loss

Let's dive into some inspiring real-life stories that highlight the transformative power of integrating mind-body practices into weight loss efforts. These case studies showcase diverse journeys towards holistic health, demonstrating how somatic practices can revolutionize your approach to wellness.

Profiles of Individuals Transforming Their Relationship with Their Bodies

1. Jenna's Journey: Embracing Body Awareness Jenna struggled with emotional eating for years, feeling disconnected from her body. Through somatic practices, she learned to tune into her hunger and fullness cues, distinguishing between emotional and physical hunger. By incorporating mindful movement and breathwork, Jenna not only lost weight but also developed a positive relationship with her body, appreciating its signals and needs.

2. Mark's Path to Mindful Eating Mark had tried numerous diets without lasting success. By integrating somatic exercises into his routine, he discovered the importance of mindfulness in eating. Practicing body awareness helped him recognize when he was starving versus eating out of stress. This shift led to sustainable weight loss and a newfound sense of control over his eating habits.

Combining Somatic Exercise, Diet Changes, and Mental Health Support

3. Sarah's Holistic Transformation Sarah faced chronic stress and weight gain. She started practicing somatic exercises and paired them with a balanced diet rich in whole foods. Additionally, she sought mental health support to address underlying stressors. This comprehensive approach not only helped her shed pounds but also enhanced her emotional well-being, creating a lasting impact on her overall health.

4. David's Comprehensive Approach. David's weight loss journey was marked by ups and downs until he adopted a holistic strategy. He combined somatic exercises with

dietary adjustments and regular therapy sessions. This trifecta approach enabled him to address both the physical and emotional aspects of weight management, leading to consistent progress and a healthier lifestyle.

The Importance of Patience, Self-Care, and a Holistic Approach

5. Lisa's Long-Term Success Lisa learned that patience and self-care are vital in her weight loss journey. Through somatic practices, she cultivated a deeper understanding of her body's needs and responses. This awareness, combined with a nutritious diet and regular self-reflection, allowed Lisa to achieve and maintain her health goals sustainably.

6. Kevin's Balanced Lifestyle
 Kevin's story underscores the power of a holistic approach. By integrating somatic exercises, he improved his body awareness and movement efficiency. Alongside these practices, he focused on eating mindfully and seeking emotional support when needed   . This balanced lifestyle helped Kevin achieve his weight loss goals while fostering a positive relationship with his body and Getting Started with Somatic Exercises

Welcome to your journey into the world of somatic exercises! This chapter is designed to help you get started with practical guidance on foundational movements, creating a personal plan, and finding resources for proper technique. Whether you're a fitness newbie or looking to add something new to your routine, somatic exercises offer a gentle, mindful way to improve your health and well-being.

CHAPTER 03

CORE SOMATIC MOVEMENTS FOR BEGINNERS

Let's dive into some basic somatic exercises that are easy to incorporate into your daily routine. These movements are accessible to everyone, regardless of fitness level.

Foundational Movements

1. **The Pelvic Tilt**

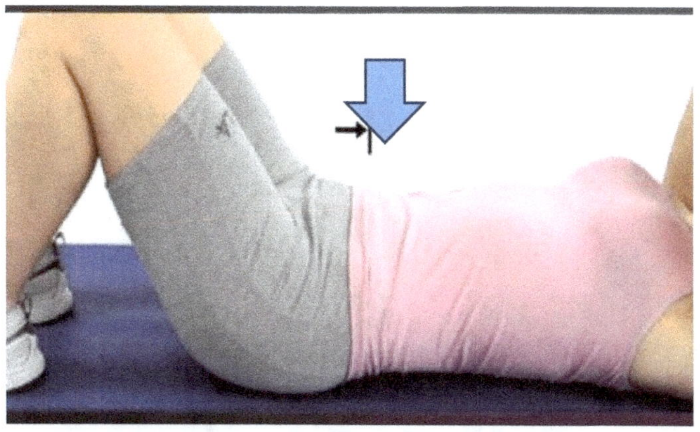

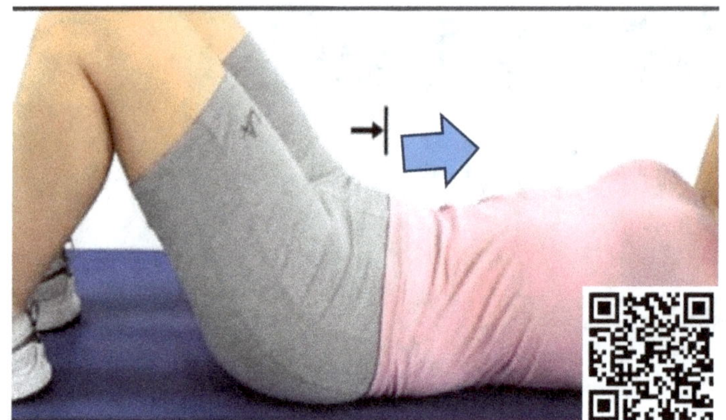

- o **Description:** Lie on your back with your knees bent and feet flat on the floor. Gently rock your pelvis back and forth, tilting it towards your belly button, then towards the floor.
- o **Benefits:** Releases lower back tension and enhances core awareness.

2. **Shoulder Rolls**

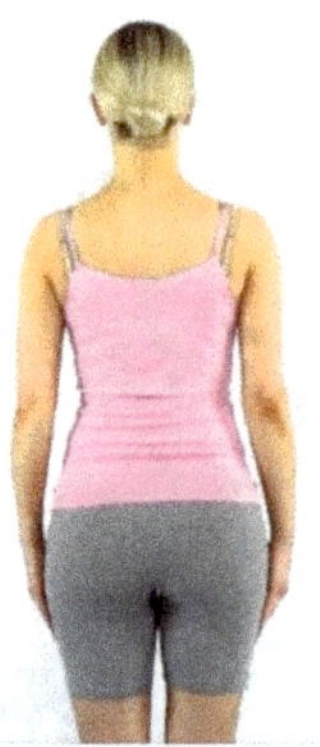

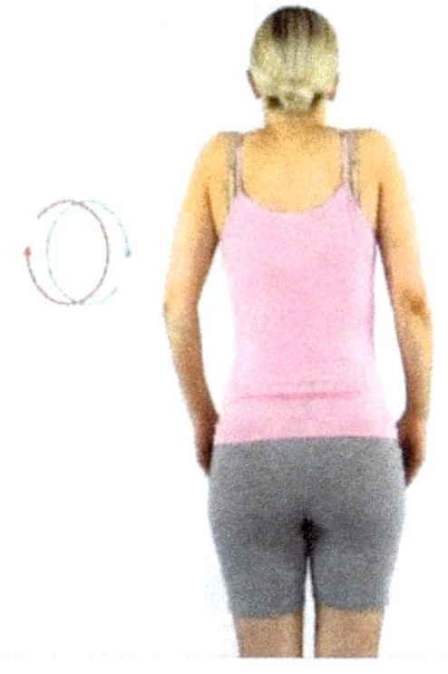

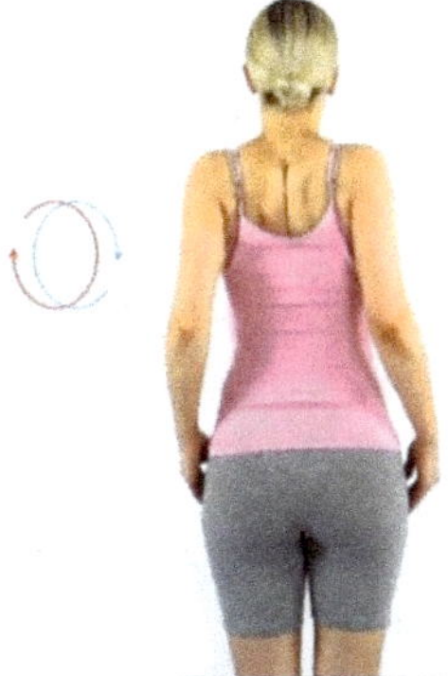

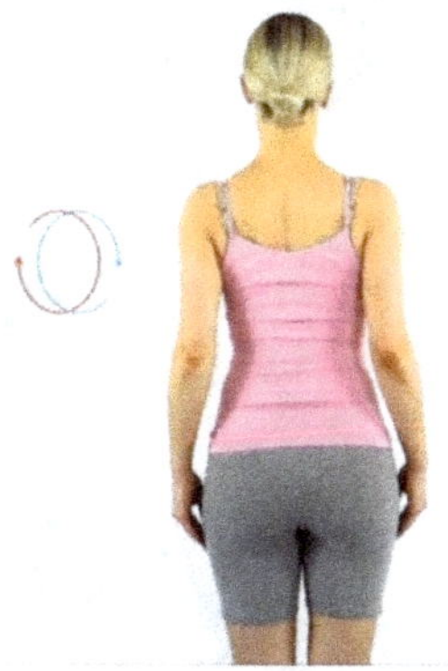

22

- o **Description:** Sit or stand comfortably. Slowly roll your shoulders up towards your ears, then back and down in a circular motion. Repeat in the opposite direction.
- o **Benefits:** Eases shoulder tension and improves upper body mobility.

3. **Cat-Cow Stretch**

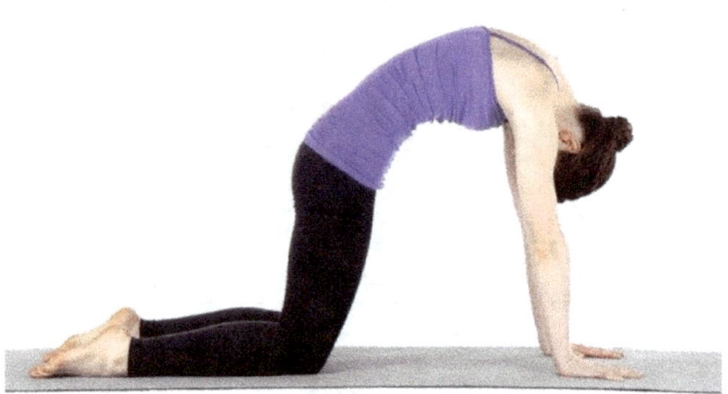

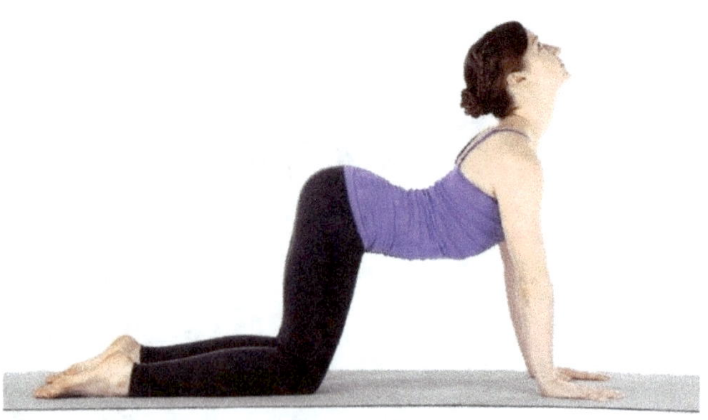

- o **Description:** Get on your hands and knees. Inhale as you arch your back (Cow), lifting your head and tailbone. Exhale as you round your back (Cat), tucking your chin and pelvis.
- o **Benefits:** Enhances spinal flexibility and relieves tension along the spine.

Approaching These Exercises with Mindfulness

When practicing somatic exercises, it's important to move mindfully. Here are a few tips:

Focus on Sensations: Pay close attention to how your body feels during each movement. Notice areas of tightness or ease.

Move Slowly: Perform each exercise slowly and gently. This allows you to fully experience the movement and its effects.

Breathe Deeply: Integrate deep, steady breathing into your routine. This helps to relax your muscles and enhance the benefits of each movement.

Simple Routines for Home Practice

Here are a few easy routines you can try at home with minimal equipment:

1. **Morning Wake-Up Routine (10 minutes)**
   - o Pelvic Tilts: 5 repetitions
   - o Shoulder Rolls: 5 rolls in each direction

- o Cat-Cow Stretch: 5 cycles
2. **Midday Refresh (5 minutes)**
   - o Shoulder Rolls: 5 rolls in each direction
   - o Seated Forward Bend: Sit with legs extended, reach towards your toes, and hold for a few breaths
   - o Gentle Twist: Sit with legs crossed, place one hand on the opposite knee, and twist gently to each side
3. **Evening Wind-Down (10 minutes)**
   - o Pelvic Tilts: 5 repetitions
   - o Cat-Cow Stretch: 5 cycles
   - o Supine Twist: Lie on your back, bring one knee towards your chest, and let it fall over to the opposite side while extending the opposite arm out

These routines can be adapted to fit your schedule and needs. The key is consistency and listening to your body.

mind.

Creating a Personalized Somatic Exercise Plan

Designing a somatic exercise plan tailored to your unique needs, goals, and lifestyle can be an exciting and transformative journey. Here's how to get started on creating a routine that fits you perfectly.

1. Assess Your Health and Goals

Understanding Your Starting Point: Begin by evaluating your current health status and fitness level. Consider any existing conditions, physical limitations, or areas of

discomfort. This will help you choose exercises that are safe and beneficial for you.

Setting Clear Goals: Identify what you want to achieve with your somatic exercise plan. Are you looking to lose weight, reduce stress, improve flexibility, or enhance overall well-being? Clear goals will guide your exercise selection and keep you motivated.

Example: If your goal is to alleviate back pain and improve posture, focus on exercises like Pelvic Tilts and Cat-Cow Stretches that target the spine and core stability.

2. Gradually Incorporate Somatic Movements

Start Slow and Steady: Introduce somatic exercises gradually into your daily routine. This prevents injury and allows your body to adapt to new movements. Begin with a few minutes each day and slowly increase the duration and intensity.

Build a Routine: Incorporate somatic exercises into activities you already do. Stretch gently while watching TV, practice mindful breathing during breaks at work, or do a short routine before bed. This integration helps form lasting habits.

Example: Start with a 5-minute morning routine of gentle stretches. As you become more comfortable, extend it to 10 minutes and include additional exercises.

Keep Your Practice Engaging and Adaptable

Variety is Key: Mix different somatic exercises to keep your routine interesting. Explore various movements that address different parts of your body and different aspects of your well-being.

Stay Attuned to Your Body: Listen to your body's signals and adjust your exercises accordingly. Some days, you may need more gentle movements, while other days, you might feel up for a more vigorous session.

Example: Alternate between a relaxing evening wind-down routine and a more energizing morning wake-up session. Keep experimenting with new exercises to find what works best for you.

4. Personalize Your Practice

Create a Plan That Fits Your Lifestyle: Design your exercise plan to fit seamlessly into your daily schedule. Choose times and settings that are convenient and comfortable for you, whether it's at home, in a park, or a quiet corner of your office.

Set Milestones and Celebrate Progress: Establish short-term milestones to track your progress and keep motivated. Celebrate your achievements, no matter how small, to stay positive and committed.

Example: Set a goal to practice somatic exercises for 15 minutes daily for a month. Reward yourself with a relaxing activity or treat when you reach your goal.

Tips for Success:

- **Stay Consistent:** Consistency is key to seeing benefits. Even on busy days, try to fit in a few minutes of somatic practice.
- **Be Patient:** Progress might be gradual. Trust the process and be patient with yourself.
- **Seek Support:** Join a class, find an exercise buddy, or use online resources for guidance and motivation.

By assessing your health, gradually incorporating exercises, keeping your practice engaging, and personalizing your plan, you can create a somatic exercise routine that not only fits your lifestyle but also evolves with your health and wellness journey.

Multimedia Resources for Correct Execution

This section introduces various multimedia aids to support correct execution and deepen understanding of somatic exercises.

1. Recommendations for Videos, Apps, and Online Communities:

- **YouTube Channels:** Search for reputable channels that specialize in somatic exercises, such as "Yoga with Adriene" or "The Feldenkrais Center."
- **Apps:** Consider apps like "Daily Yoga," "Glo," or "Somatic Movement Center" for guided sessions.
- **Online Communities:** Join forums or social media groups such as Reddit's r/yoga or Facebook groups dedicated to somatic practices.

2. Utilizing These Resources Effectively:

- **Refining Technique:** Follow step-by-step instructional videos to ensure correct form and avoid injury.
- **Staying Motivated:** Use apps with progress tracking and reminders to maintain consistency.
- **Engaging with Communities:** Participate in online discussions to share experiences, seek advice, and find encouragement.

3. Critical Assessment of Resources:

- **Align with Wellness Philosophies:** Ensure the content aligns with your personal health beliefs and goals.
- **Evaluate Instructors' Credentials:** Check the qualifications of instructors to ensure they provide accurate and safe guidance.
- **User Reviews:** Read reviews and testimonials to gauge the effectiveness and reliability of the resources.

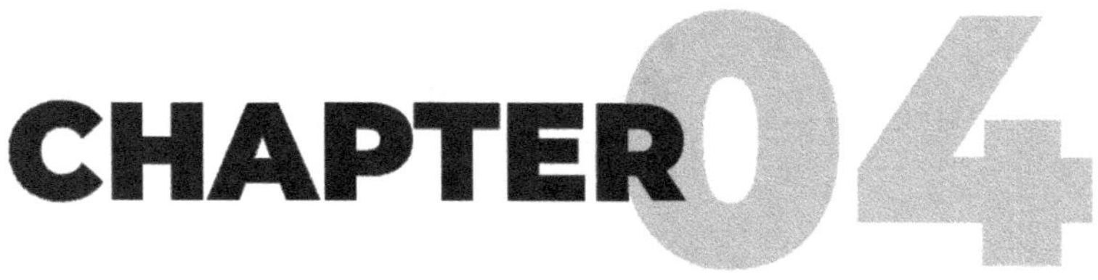

CHAPTER 04

INTEGRATING DIET AND NUTRITION

Transitioning our focus to how diet and nutrition support somatic exercises and overall wellness, this chapter provides practical advice on meal planning, managing cravings, and understanding nutritional needs.

Nutritional Foundations for Supporting Somatic Exercise

A balanced diet is crucial for complementing somatic practice, aiding weight loss, and enhancing physical health. Here's what you need to know:

The Role of Macronutrients and Micronutrients

1. **Macronutrients:**
   - **Proteins:** Essential for muscle repair and recovery. Include lean meats, beans, and nuts in your diet.
   - **Carbohydrates:** Provide energy for your workouts. Opt for whole grains, fruits, and vegetables.

- o **Fats:** Necessary for hormone production and cell function. Focus on healthy fats from avocados, nuts, and olive oil.

2. **Micronutrients:**
   - o **Vitamins and Minerals:** Vital for overall health and bodily functions. Ensure a varied diet rich in colorful fruits and vegetables to meet your micronutrient needs.

Hydration and Performance

Hydration is vital to maintaining bodily awareness and performance during somatic exercises. Water helps regulate body temperature, lubricate joints and transport nutrients. Aim to drink water consistently throughout the day, especially before and after your workouts.

Pre- and Post-Exercise Meals

1. **Pre-Exercise:**
   - o **Light Snack:** Consume a small meal or snack that includes both carbohydrates and protein about 30 minutes to an hour before exercising. For example, a banana with a tablespoon of almond butter.
2. **Post-Exercise:**
   - o **Recovery Meal:** Within an hour after exercising, have a balanced meal that includes protein and carbohydrates to replenish energy stores and support muscle recovery. For example, a grilled chicken salad with quinoa and a variety of vegetables.

By understanding and applying these nutritional principles, you can optimize your somatic exercise routine, supporting both your weight loss and overall wellness goals.

Meal Planning and Prep for Busy Lifestyles

Balancing a busy lifestyle with healthy eating can be challenging, but with the right strategies, it becomes manageable. This segment provides comprehensive tips for incorporating healthful eating into your schedule, emphasizing the importance of preparation and planning.

Time-Saving Tips and Tricks for Meal Prep

1. **Simple Recipes:**
   - **Choose Quick Recipes:** Opt for recipes that are quick to prepare and require minimal ingredients.
     - **Example:** A stir-fry with mixed vegetables and lean protein.
   - **One-Pot Meals:** Reduce cleanup time by preparing meals that use only one pot or pan.
     - **Example:** A quinoa and vegetable skillet.
2. **Prep Ahead:**
   - **Dedicated Prep Time:** Set aside a few hours once a week to prepare meals for the days ahead.
     - **Example:** Wash and chop vegetables, cook grains and proteins in bulk.
   - **Portion Control:** Divide prepared food into individual portions for easy grab-and-go options.
     - **Example:** Store salads in mason jars or meal components in stackable containers.

3. **Utilize Kitchen Gadgets:**
    - **Slow Cooker:** Prepare large batches of food with minimal hands-on time.
        - **Example:** Use a slow cooker to prepare a large batch of soup while you're at work.
    - **Instant Pot:** Speed up cooking times for beans, grains, and meats.
        - **Example:** Cook a whole chicken or a pot of chili in under an hour.
    - **Blender:** Quickly prepare smoothies, sauces, and soups.
        - **Example:** Blend a green smoothie for a quick breakfast.

Creating a Flexible Meal Plan

1. **Plan for Versatility:**
    - **Base Ingredients:** Create meals that can be easily modified with different toppings or sides.
        - **Example:** Prepare a base like quinoa or rice that can be paired with different proteins and veggies.
    - **Mix and Match:** Use ingredients that can be repurposed in various dishes.
        - **Example:** Cooked chicken can be used in salads, wraps, or stir-fries.
2. **Adapt to Changes:**
    - **Keep Staples on Hand:** Have ingredients available that can quickly adjust to changes in appetite or schedule.
        - **Example:** Have canned beans, frozen vegetables, and pre-cooked chicken available.

- o **Flexible Recipes:** Choose recipes that allow for substitutions based on what's available.
    - **Example:** A vegetable curry that can be made with whatever veggies you have on hand.

3. **Balanced Meals:**
    - o **Nutrition Focus:** Ensure each meal contains a mix of protein, carbs, and fats.
        - **Example:** A salad with mixed greens, grilled chicken, nuts, and a light vinaigrette.
    - o **Snack Prep:** Prepare healthy snacks to prevent unhealthy eating.
        - **Example:** Cut up veggies with hummus or portion out nuts and fruit.

Batch Cooking, Shopping Lists, and Organizational Tools

1. **Batch Cooking:**
    - o **Large Portions:** Cook large portions of staples like grains, proteins, and vegetables.
        - **Example:** Prepare a big pot of chili or a large tray of roasted vegetables.
    - o **Freezing Meals:** Freeze portions for future use to save time on busy days.
        - **Example:** Freeze soups, stews, and casseroles in single -serving containers.

2. **Shopping Lists:**
    - o **Weekly Planning:** Plan your shopping list based on your weekly meal plan.
        - **Example:** Create a list of ingredients needed for each meal to avoid multiple trips to the store.

- o **Stick to the List:** Avoid impulse buys and ensure you have all the necessary ingredients.
  - **Example:** List items by category (produce, dairy, proteins) to streamline your shopping.

3. **Organizational Tools:**
   - o **Meal Planning Apps:** Use apps or planners to track your meal plans and grocery lists.
     - **Example:** Apps like Mealime or Yummly can provide recipes and generate shopping lists.
   - o **Pantry Organization:** Keep a well-organized pantry with labeled containers for easy access.
     - **Example:** Store grains, nuts, and seeds in clear, labeled containers.
   - o **Calendar Integration:** Use a calendar to schedule meal prep times and plan meals.
     - **Example:** Sync your meal plan with your digital calendar to stay on track.

Easy Recipes (Bonus)

1. Quinoa and Vegetable Stir-Fry

Ingredients:

- 1 cup quinoa
- 2 cups vegetable broth
- 1 tablespoon olive oil
- 1 bell pepper, chopped
- 1 zucchini, chopped
- 1 carrot, julienned
- 1 cup broccoli florets
- 2 cloves garlic, minced
- 2 tablespoons soy sauce

- 1 tablespoon sesame seeds

Instructions:

1. Cook quinoa in vegetable broth according to package instructions.
2. In a large skillet, heat olive oil over medium heat. Add garlic and sauté until fragrant.
3. Add bell pepper, zucchini, carrot, and broccoli to the skillet. Stir-fry until vegetables are tender.
4. Add cooked quinoa and soy sauce to the skillet. Stir well to combine.
5. Sprinkle with sesame seeds before serving.

2. Slow Cooker Chicken and Vegetable Soup

Ingredients:

- 1-pound boneless, skinless chicken breasts
- 4 cups chicken broth
- 1 cup diced tomatoes
- 2 carrots, sliced
- 2 celery stalks, sliced
- 1 onion, chopped
- 2 cloves garlic, minced
- 1 teaspoon dried thyme
- 1 teaspoon dried basil
- Salt and pepper to taste
- 2 cups spinach leaves

Instructions:

1. Place chicken breasts, chicken broth, diced tomatoes, carrots, celery, onion, garlic, thyme, and basil into the slow cooker.
2. Season with salt and pepper. Stir to combine.

3. Cook on low for 6-8 hours or on high for 3-4 hours.
4. Remove the chicken, shred it with a fork, and return it to the slow cooker.
5. Add spinach leaves and cook for an additional 10 minutes until wilted.
6. Serve hot and enjoy.

CHAPTER 05

SOMATIC PRACTICES FOR STRESS AND ANXIETY RELIEF

Stress and anxiety are pervasive issues that can profoundly impact both physical and emotional health. Somatic exercises offer a holistic approach to alleviating these conditions by utilizing body awareness to foster emotional health. This section details specific somatic practices designed to release tension, regulate the nervous system, and break the cycle of stress-related thought patterns.

Exercises for Releasing Muscular Tension and Restoring Physiological Balance

Muscular tension is a common physical manifestation of stress and anxiety. Releasing this tension can help restore physiological balance and mitigate stress responses.

Progressive Muscle Relaxation (PMR):

[Progressive Muscle Relaxation](#)

Description: PMR involves tensing and then slowly releasing different muscle groups in the body.
Method:
- o Find a comfortable position, either sitting or lying down.
- o Start with your feet, tense the muscles tightly for 5-10 seconds, then release and relax for 20-30 seconds.
- o Move progressively up through your body: calves, thighs, abdomen, chest, arms, and face.

Benefits: Reduces muscle tension, enhances body awareness, and promotes relaxation.

Body Scan Meditation:

[Body Scan Meditation](#)

Description: This practice involves mentally scanning your body for areas of tension or discomfort.
Method:
- o Lie down or sit comfortably with your eyes closed.
- o Starting from your toes, slowly bring your attention to each part of your body, noticing any sensations.
- o Spend a few moments on each area, consciously relaxing any tension you find.

Benefits: Increases bodily awareness, reduces tension, and fosters a deep sense of relaxation.

Gentle Stretching:

Gentle Stretching:

Description: Incorporating gentle stretching can help release physical tension and promote relaxation.
Method:
- o Perform stretches targeting major muscle groups, such as neck rolls, shoulder shrugs, and hamstring stretches.
- o Hold each stretch for 15-30 seconds, breathing deeply.

Benefits: Improves flexibility, reduces muscle tightness, and enhances overall physical comfort.

2. The Role of Breath Work in Regulating the Nervous System

Breathwork is a powerful tool for regulating the nervous system and inducing a state of calm. Different techniques can activate the parasympathetic nervous system, which helps counteract the stress response.

Diaphragmatic Breathing:

Diaphragmatic Breathing

Description: Also known as belly breathing, this technique emphasizes deep breathing from the diaphragm.
Method:
- o Sit or lie down in a comfortable position.
- o Place one hand on your chest and the other on your abdomen.

- o Inhale deeply through your nose, allowing your abdomen to rise while keeping your chest relatively still.
- o Exhale slowly through your mouth, feeling your abdomen fall.

Benefits: Reduces stress hormones, lowers blood pressure, and promotes relaxation.

Box Breathing:

[Box Breathing](#)

Description: A technique involving equal parts inhalation, holding, exhalation, and holding the breath again.

Method:
- o Inhale deeply for a count of four.
- o Hold your breath for a count of four.
- o Exhale slowly for a count of four.
- o Hold your breath again for a count of four.
- o Repeat the cycle several times.

Benefits: Enhances focus, reduces anxiety, and promotes a sense of calm.

Alternate Nostril Breathing:

[Alternate Nostril Breathing](#)

Description: This technique balances the flow of air through both nostrils, helping to regulate the nervous system.

Method:
- o Sit comfortably and use your right thumb to close your right nostril.
- o Inhale deeply through your left nostril.

- o Close your left nostril with your right ring finger and hold your breath briefly.
- o Open your right nostril and exhale slowly through it.
- o Inhale through your right nostril, close it, and exhale through your left nostril.
- o Repeat the cycle for several minutes.

Benefits: Balances the nervous system, enhances mental clarity, and reduces stress.

3. Using Movement to Break the Cycle of Stress-Related Thought Patterns

Movement can be an effective way to break the cycle of stress-related thought patterns and behaviors, promoting a sense of well-being and mental clarity.

Mindful Walking:

[Mindful Walking](#)

Description: Walking with a focus on the present moment and bodily sensations.
Method:
- o Find a quiet place where you can walk undisturbed.
- o Stroll, paying attention to the sensations in your feet and legs.
- o Notice your surroundings, the sounds, and the rhythm of your breath.

Benefits: Reduces stress, improves mood, and enhances mindfulness.

Yoga:

Yoga:

Description: A practice that combines physical postures, breath control, and meditation.
Method:
- o Practice gentle yoga poses such as Child's Pose, Cat-Cow, and Downward Dog.
- o Focus on your breath and the sensations in your body as you move through each pose.

Benefits: Improves flexibility, reduces stress, and promotes overall well-being.

Tai Chi:

Tai Chi

Description: A form of martial arts known for its slow, flowing movements and focus on breath control.
Method:
- o Learn basic Tai Chi forms and practice them regularly.
- o Focus on smooth, deliberate movements and deep, rhythmic breathing.

Benefits: Enhances physical and mental balance, reduces anxiety, and promotes relaxation.

By integrating these somatic practices into your daily routine, you can effectively manage stress and anxiety. These techniques help release physical tension, regulate the nervous system, and interrupt stress-related thought patterns, contributing to a greater sense of well-being and emotional health.

Building Resilience Against Emotional Eating

Emotional eating can be a challenging habit to break, but with the right strategies, you can develop healthier coping mechanisms. Here's how to address the root causes of emotional eating and manage cravings and stress holistically.

Identifying Emotional Triggers and Creating Alternative Responses

Identify Triggers:

> **Keep a Journal:** Write down when and why you feel the urge to eat emotionally. Look for patterns in your emotions and behaviors.
> - **Example:** Note if stress at work leads you to snack more in the evenings.

Create a Toolkit:

> **Alternative Responses:** Develop a list of activities to do instead of eating when you're emotional.
> - **Examples:** Go for a walk, call a friend, practice deep breathing, or engage in a hobby.

2. The Significance of Self-Compassion and Patience

Self-Compassion:

> **Be Kind to Yourself:** Understand that emotional eating is a common struggle, and be gentle with yourself as you work to change.

- **Example:** Instead of feeling guilty after emotional eating, acknowledge the slip-up and plan to try a different coping mechanism next time.

Patience:

Allow Time for Change: Changing habits takes time. Celebrate small victories and be patient with your progress.
- **Example:** If you manage to use an alternative coping mechanism once a week, that's a success worth recognizing.

3. Community Support Options

Group Therapy:

Find Support: Join a group therapy session to share experiences and learn from others facing similar challenges.
- **Example:** Look for local or online support groups focused on emotional eating.

Somatic Exercise Classes:

Engage with Others: Participate in classes like yoga or Tai Chi, where you can build a community and receive encouragement.
- **Example:** Join a weekly yoga class to connect with others and reduce stress.

ADVANCED SOMATIC EXERCISES FOR WEIGHT LOSS

Welcome to the next level of your somatic exercise journey! This chapter focuses on advanced techniques to intensify your weight loss efforts. We'll highlight the importance of progression and adapting exercises to suit your physical capabilities.

Introduction to Dynamic Somatic Exercises

As you advance in your somatic practice, incorporating more dynamic exercises can help accelerate weight loss and enhance overall fitness. Here are some exercises designed for intermediate to advanced individuals:

Somatic Flow Sequences:

[Somatic Flow Sequences](#)

Description: These sequences combine multiple movements into a continuous flow, challenging coordination and stamina.
Example: A sequence might include a series of spinal rolls, hip circles, and dynamic stretches performed fluidly.

Advanced Core Work:

[Advanced Core Work](#)

Description: Engage deeper core muscles with more complex movements.
Example: Try plank variations, such as side planks with leg lifts or dynamic planks where you transition from forearms to hands.

Full-Body Integrative Movements:

[Full-Body Integrative Movements](#)

Description: These exercises involve multiple muscle groups, promoting functional strength.
Example: Incorporate exercises like Turkish get-ups or full-body somatic flows that integrate balance, strength, and flexibility.

Methods to Safely Increase Intensity

Increasing the intensity of your somatic exercises should be done gradually to avoid injury and ensure sustainable progress. Here are some methods to safely up the ante:

1. Gradual Progression:

Incremental Increases: Slowly increase the duration or intensity of each exercise.
Example: If you're used to a 30-second plank, try extending it to 45 seconds over a few weeks.

2. Listen to Your Body:

Body Signals: Pay attention to your body's feedback. Discomfort is normal, but sharp pain is a signal to stop.
Example: If you feel strain in your lower back during an exercise, modify the movement or take a break.

3. Proper Warm-Up and Cool-Down:

Warm-Up: Always start with a thorough warm-up to prepare your muscles and joints.
Example: Begin with gentle stretches and light aerobic activity.
Cool-Down: End with a cool-down to aid recovery.
Example: Finish with deep breathing and slow, static stretches.

Diverse Routines for Comprehensive Workouts

To ensure a well-rounded fitness regimen, incorporate routines that target different muscle groups. This approach not only promotes balanced muscle development but also keeps your workouts interesting.

1. **Upper Body Focus:**

Upper Body Focus

Routine Example: Combine shoulder rolls, arm circles, and dynamic planks to engage the shoulders, chest, and arms.

Advanced Moves: Add resistance bands or light weights to increase difficulty.

2. **Lower Body Focus:**

[Lower Body Focus](#)

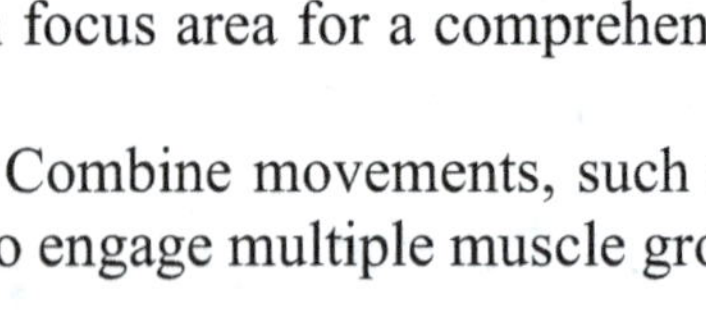

Routine Example: Include hip openers, lunges, and squats to target the hips, thighs, and glutes.

Advanced Moves: Try single-leg exercises or plyometric movements like jump squats.

3. **Core Strength Focus:**

[Core Strength Focus](#)

Routine Example: Perform a mix of core-engaging exercises like leg raises, dynamic planks, and twisting motions.

Advanced Moves: Incorporate stability balls or balance boards to challenge your core further.

4. **Full-Body Integration:**

[Full-Body Integrative Movements](#)

Routine Example: Design a circuit that includes exercises from each focus area for a comprehensive session.

Advanced Moves: Combine movements, such as a lunge with a twist, to engage multiple muscle groups simultaneously.

The Role of Intensity and Progression
Understanding the critical role that workout intensity and progressive overload play is essential for advancing weight loss and physical fitness through somatic practices. This section explores techniques to safely increase workout intensity, the science behind these principles, and how to create a balanced workout plan that includes rest and recovery.

Techniques to Progressively Overload the Body Safely

1. Gradual Increase in Exercise Difficulty:
 Description: Slowly increase the complexity or duration of your exercises to challenge your body.
 Methods:
- **Duration:** Extend the time you spend on each exercise.
  - **Example:** If you typically perform a somatic flow sequence for 10 minutes, increase it to 12 minutes.
- **Repetitions:** Increase the number of repetitions for each movement.
  - **Example:** If you do 10 repetitions of a dynamic plank, gradually increase to 15.
- **Resistance:** Add light weights or resistance bands to your routine.
  - **Example:** Incorporate a resistance band into your squats or lunges to add more challenge.

3. Variation in Exercises:

[Variation in Exercises](#)

Description: Introducing new exercises regularly prevents plateaus and continuously challenges your muscles.

Methods:

- o **New Movements:** Add different somatic exercises to your routine.

    Example: Try new variations of core exercises, like incorporating a stability ball for planks.

- o **Exercise Combinations:** Combine multiple exercises into a complex movement.

    Example: Combine a squat with an overhead press to engage more muscle groups.

The Science Behind Workout Intensity

1. Correlation with Fat Loss:

High-Intensity Training: Engaging in high-intensity somatic exercises increases calorie burn and promotes fat loss.

- o **Science:** High-intensity exercises elevate your heart rate and metabolic rate, leading to greater energy expenditure both during and after the workout.

- o **Example:** Incorporating intervals of high-intensity somatic movements, like fast-paced dynamic stretches, can boost fat loss.

2. Muscle Building:

Progressive Overload Principle: Gradually increasing the stress on your muscles leads to hypertrophy (muscle growth).

- o **Science:** When muscles are exposed to greater resistance or more challenging exercises, they adapt by growing stronger and larger.

o **Example:** Gradually increasing the weight or resistance in your somatic exercises stimulates muscle growth.

3. Benefits of Varied Intensity:
Metabolic Adaptation: Varying the intensity of your workouts prevents your body from adapting too quickly, maintaining a higher metabolic rate.
o **Example:** Alternate between high-intensity and moderate-intensity workouts throughout the week to keep your metabolism active.

Creating a Balanced Workout Plan
1. Incorporating Rest and Recovery:
Importance of Rest: Allowing your body time to recover is crucial for muscle repair and growth, as well as preventing injury.
o **Methods:**
Rest Days: Schedule regular rest days in your workout plan.
Example: Include at least one or two rest days per week where you engage in light activities like walking or gentle stretching.
Active Recovery: On lighter days, engage in low-intensity activities that promote blood flow and recovery without taxing your muscles.
Example: Perform gentle yoga or a slow-paced walk.

2. Balanced Routine:
Variety of Exercises: Ensure your workout plan includes exercises targeting different muscle groups and aspects of fitness (strength, flexibility, endurance).

o **Methods:**

Weekly Schedule: Design a weekly schedule that balances intense workouts with lighter sessions and rest periods.

Example:

Monday: High-intensity somatic flow
Tuesday: Moderate-intensity core and balance work
Wednesday: Rest or gentle yoga
Thursday: High-intensity interval training (HIIT) with somatic movements
Friday: Low-intensity flexibility and stretching
Saturday: Full-body somatic workout
Sunday: Rest or active recovery

3. Monitoring Progress:

Track Your Workouts: Keep a log of your exercises, intensity, duration, and how you feel after each session.

o **Example:** Use a fitness journal or app to record your workouts and progress.

Adjust as Needed: Based on your progress and how your body responds, adjust your plan to continue challenging yourself.

Example: If you notice improvements in strength and endurance, gradually increase the intensity or add new exercises

Caution and Adaptation for Physical Limitations

Adapting somatic exercises to accommodate individual physical limitations is essential to ensure a safe and effective workout experience. Here are strategies for modifications, the importance of body awareness, and the value of consulting healthcare professionals.

Modifications to Common Somatic Exercises

For individuals with specific health conditions or injuries, modifying exercises can make somatic practices accessible and safe.

Lower Back Pain:

> **Modification:** Avoid exercises that put a strain on the lower back, such as deep forward bends or heavy lifting.
> - o **Example:** Replace traditional forward bends with supported forward folds using a chair or bolster.
> - o **Somatic Alternative:** Gentle pelvic tilts while lying on your back can help strengthen the core without stressing the lower back.

Knee Issues:

> **Modification:** Reduce stress on the knees by avoiding deep squats or lunges.
> - o **Example:** Perform half squats or use a chair for support during lunges.
> - o **Somatic Alternative:** Seated leg lifts and extensions can strengthen the quadriceps and support knee health without added strain.

Shoulder Injuries:

> **Modification:** Limit overhead movements and heavy lifting.
> - o **Example:** Instead of overhead presses, try lateral raises with light weights or resistance bands.

- o **Somatic Alternative:** Shoulder rolls and gentle arm circles can improve mobility and reduce tension without aggravating injuries.

Arthritis:

Modification: Avoid high-impact or repetitive stress activities.
- o **Example:** Replace running or high-impact aerobics with low-impact exercises like swimming or cycling.
- o **Somatic Alternative:** Gentle yoga or Tai Chi movements can enhance flexibility and reduce joint stiffness.

Importance of Listening to Your Body

Body Awareness:

Pay Attention: Always listen to your body's signals during exercise. Discomfort is normal, but sharp pain indicates you should stop.
- o **Tip:** If you feel pain during an exercise, modify the movement or take a break.
- o **Example:** If lunges cause knee pain, switch to a supported variation or focus on leg stretches instead.

Adjusting Intensity:

Start Slow: Begin with low-intensity exercises and gradually increase as your strength and endurance improve.
- o **Tip:** Monitor your progress and adjust the intensity of your workouts based on how your body responds.

o **Example:** If you feel fatigued after a high-intensity workout, incorporate more rest days or switch to moderate-intensity exercises.

Consultation with Healthcare Professionals

Personalized Exercise Plans:

Seek Professional Advice: Before starting a new exercise regimen, especially if you have health conditions or injuries, consult a healthcare professional.

o **Tip:** Work with a physical therapist, physician, or certified trainer who can tailor a somatic exercise plan to your needs.

o **Example:** A physical therapist can recommend specific exercises that support recovery from injury and prevent further issues.

Regular Check-Ins:

Ongoing Support: Regularly check in with your healthcare provider to assess your progress and make necessary adjustments to your exercise plan.

o **Tip:** Keep a log of your exercises and any discomfort or pain experienced, and share this with your healthcare provider.

o **Example:** If you notice increased pain or discomfort, discuss this with your healthcare provider to adjust your routine appropriately.

CHAPTER 07

PRINCIPLES OF MINDFUL EATING

Mindful eating is a transformative approach that helps reduce overeating and fosters a healthy relationship with food. By focusing on the present moment and tuning into your body's needs, you can make more conscious choices and enjoy your meals more fully.

The Significance of Eating Slowly and with Intention

1. Enhanced Digestion and Satisfaction:

Eating Slowly:
- o **Practice:** Take smaller bites, chew thoroughly, and put your utensils down between bites.
- o **Benefit:** This allows your body more time to process food, leading to better digestion and increased feelings of fullness.

Eating with Intention:
- o **Practice:** Focus on the flavors, textures, and aromas of your food. Engage all your senses.

- o **Benefit:** This enhances the overall eating experience and can lead to greater satisfaction with smaller amounts of food.

Using Mindfulness to Recognize Hunger Cues

1. Distinguishing Emotional from Physical Hunger:

Emotional Hunger:
- o **Characteristics:** Sudden urgent cravings, often for specific comfort foods, not satisfied by a full stomach.
- o **Mindfulness Practice:** Pause and ask yourself if you are truly hungry or if you are eating to address an emotion like stress or boredom.

Physical Hunger:
- o **Characteristics:** Gradual onset, open to a variety of foods, satisfied by eating.
- o **Mindfulness Practice:** Pay attention to bodily sensations like stomach growling or low energy levels as indicators of true hunger.

Creating an Eating Environment that Fosters Attentiveness and Enjoyment

1. Setting the Scene:

Reduce Distractions:
- o **Practice:** Turn off the TV, put away smartphones, and focus solely on your meal.
- o **Benefit:** This helps you fully engage with your food and notice when you are satisfied.

Create a Pleasant Atmosphere:
- o **Practice:** Set the table nicely, play soft music, or eat in a peaceful environment.
- o **Benefit:** A pleasant setting can make meals more enjoyable and encourage slower, more mindful eating.

Listening to Your Body's Hunger and Fullness Cues

Learning to accurately interpret and respond to your body's hunger and fullness cues is key to preventing overeating and maintaining a healthy relationship with food.

Identifying True Hunger Signals

1. Recognizing True Hunger:

Hunger Signals:
- o **Physical Indicators:** Growling stomach, light headedness, low energy.
- o **Mindfulness Practice:** Before eating, rate your hunger on a scale from 1 to 10 to determine if you are truly hungry.

Habit and Trigger Recognition:
- o **Common Triggers:** Time of day, social settings, emotions.
- o **Mindfulness Practice:** Notice patterns and question whether you are eating out of habit or actual hunger.

Stopping at the Point of Satisfaction

1. Tips for Recognizing Fullness:

Eat Slowly:
- o **Practice:** Slow down and chew each bite thoroughly.
- o **Benefit:** This allows time for satiety signals to reach your brain.

Mid-Meal Check-In:
- o **Practice:** Pause halfway through your meal and assess your hunger level.
- o **Benefit:** This helps you determine if you are still hungry or if you can stop eating.

The Role of Journaling and Reflection

1. Food Journaling:

Practice: Keep a journal of what you eat, your hunger levels before and after eating, and any emotions you experience.
- o **Benefit:** This can help you identify patterns and triggers, making it easier to understand your body's signals.

Reflection:
- o **Practice:** Reflect on your eating experiences, noting what worked well and what could be improved.
- o **Benefit:** This fosters greater self-awareness and helps you make more mindful choices in the future.

By adopting these principles of mindful eating, you can reduce overeating, enhance your digestion and satisfaction,

and develop a healthier, more enjoyable relationship with food. Through practices like eating slowly, recognizing actual hunger cues, and creating a mindful eating environment, you can support your overall well-being and weight management goals.

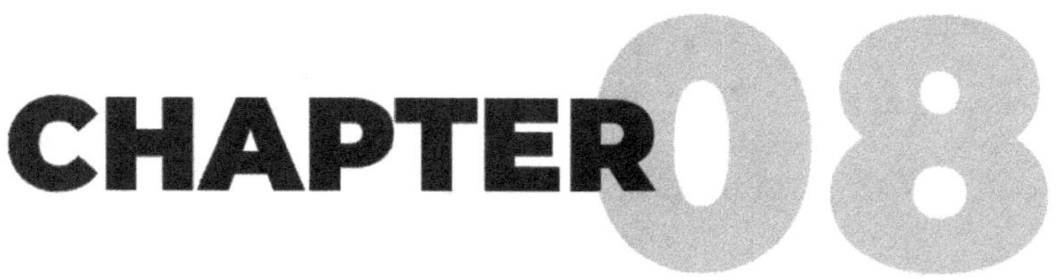

CHAPTER 08

OVERCOMING OBSTACLES AND SETTING REALISTIC GOALS

Embarking on a journey towards holistic weight loss is filled with challenges, but understanding and addressing these obstacles can pave the way for sustainable progress. This chapter dives into common barriers and offers strategies for setting realistic, achievable goals.

Common Challenges in Holistic Weight Loss Journeys

Psychological and Emotional Barriers

1. Stress and Its Impact:

> **Description:** Chronic stress can lead to hormonal imbalances, increased appetite, and cravings for unhealthy foods.
>
> **Strategies:**
> - **Mindfulness Practices:** Incorporate techniques like meditation, yoga, or deep breathing to manage stress.

- o **Stress Management Plans:** Develop a personal plan that includes regular physical activity, adequate sleep, and hobbies that promote relaxation.

2. Emotional Eating:

Description: Using food as a coping mechanism for emotions like sadness, boredom, or anxiety.
Strategies:
- o **Identify Triggers:** Keep a journal to track emotional eating episodes and identify patterns.
- o **Alternative Coping Mechanisms:** Replace eating with other activities such as going for a walk, reading, or engaging in a hobby.
- o **Mindful Eating:** Practice mindful eating to distinguish between physical hunger and emotional hunger.

3. Self-Doubt and Negative Self-Talk:

Description: Lack of confidence and negative self-perception can derail weight loss efforts.
Strategies:
- o **Positive Affirmations:** Use positive affirmations and self-talk to build self-confidence.
- o **Support Networks:** Seek support from friends, family, or support groups to encourage and motivate.
- o **Professional Help:** Consider therapy or counseling to address deep-seated issues and build a positive self-image.

Physical Challenges

1. Injuries and Chronic Conditions:

Description: Physical limitations due to injuries or chronic health issues can hinder exercise routines.
Strategies:
- **Adapted Exercises:** Work with a fitness professional to adapt exercises that accommodate your condition.
- **Rehabilitation:** Engage in physical therapy to recover from injuries and improve functionality.
- **Low-Impact Activities:** Focus on low-impact exercises such as swimming, cycling, or chair yoga to stay active without exacerbating issues.

2. Initial Lack of Fitness:

Description: Starting a fitness journey can be daunting, especially with low initial fitness levels.
Strategies:
- **Gradual Progression:** Start with short, low-intensity workouts and gradually increase duration and intensity.
- **Set Small Goals:** Set small, achievable goals to build confidence and momentum.
- **Celebrate Milestones:** Celebrate small achievements to stay motivated and track progress.

Social and Environmental Obstacles

1. Unsupportive Social Circles:

Description: Lack of support from friends and family can make it challenging to stick to healthy habits.
Strategies:
- **Communicate Needs:** Clearly communicate your goals and needs to your social circle.
- **Find Like-Minded Individuals:** Join clubs, groups, or online communities with similar health goals.
- **Lead by Example:** Inspire others by sharing your journey and successes.

2. Lack of Accessibility to Healthy Options:

Description: Limited access to healthy foods or safe places to exercise can impede progress.
Strategies:
- **Plan and Prepare:** Plan meals ahead of time and prepare healthy snacks to avoid unhealthy choices.
- **Utilize Resources:** Look for local resources like farmers' markets, community gardens, or public parks.
- **Home Workouts:** Use online resources for at-home workouts if access to a gym is limited.

3. Busy Lifestyle:

Description: A hectic schedule can make it hard to prioritize health and wellness.

Strategies:

- o **Time Management:** Schedule workouts and meal prep sessions just like any other important appointment.
- o **Efficient Workouts:** Choose quick, effective workouts such as high-intensity interval training (HIIT) or 10-minute routines.
- o **Healthy Convenience Foods:** Stock up on healthy convenience foods like pre-washed salads, frozen vegetables, and lean proteins.

By identifying these common challenges and employing targeted strategies, you can overcome obstacles and make steady, sustainable progress on your holistic weight loss journey. Setting realistic goals is the next crucial step in ensuring long-term success and well-being.

Strategies for Staying Motivated and Accountable

Staying motivated and accountable is crucial for achieving weight loss goals. This section explores effective techniques and approaches to maintain your commitment and drive throughout your weight loss journey.

Setting Up a Support System

1. Involving Friends and Family:

Description: Having a support system can provide encouragement, motivation, and accountability.

Strategies:

- o **Share Your Goals:** Let your friends and family know about your weight loss goals so they can support you.
- o **Workout Buddies:** Partner with a friend or family member for regular workouts to make

exercise more enjoyable and hold each other accountable.

- o **Healthy Activities:** Plan healthy activities with loved ones, such as cooking nutritious meals together or going for group hikes.

2. Joining Support Groups:

Description: Being part of a support group can offer a sense of community and shared experience.

Strategies:

- o **Online Communities:** Join online forums or social media groups focused on weight loss and healthy living.
- o **Local Groups:** Look for local support groups or weight loss programs where you can share experiences and tips.
- o **Regular Meetings:** Attend regular meetings or check-ins to stay engaged and motivated.

Using Tools and Apps for Tracking Progress

1. Tracking progress:

Description: Monitoring your progress helps you stay focused and recognize your achievements.

Strategies:

- o **Fitness Apps:** Use fitness apps like MyFitnessPal, Fitbit, or Lose It! to log your workouts, track your calorie intake, and monitor your progress.
- o **Progress Photos:** Take regular photos to track your transformation visually.
- o **Measurements:** Keep track of body measurements (waist, hips, chest) along with weight to see comprehensive progress.

2. Setting Reminders:

Description: Regular reminders can help keep you on track with your exercise and mindful eating practices.

Strategies:

- o **Calendar Alerts:** Set reminders on your phone or calendar for workouts and meal prep sessions.
- o **App Notifications:** Enable notifications on your fitness apps to remind you to log meals, drink water, and exercise.
- o **Sticky Notes:** Place sticky notes with motivational messages or reminders in visible places, such as your bathroom mirror or refrigerator.

Revisiting and Adjusting Goals

1. Regular Goal Review:

Description: Regularly reviewing and adjusting your goals can help maintain motivation and ensure they remain realistic and achievable.

Strategies:

- o **Monthly Check-Ins:** Set aside time each month to review your progress and adjust your goals as needed.
- o **SMART Goals:** Ensure your goals are Specific, Measurable, Achievable, Relevant, and Time-bound.
- o **Celebrate Milestones:** Celebrate your achievements, no matter how small, to stay motivated.

2. Adapting to Changes:

Description: Flexibility is important as your circumstances and abilities evolve.

Strategies:

- o **Listen to Your Body:** Adjust your workout intensity and diet based on how your body feels and responds.
- o **Life Events:** Be prepared to modify your goals and routines to accommodate changes in your life, such as a new job or a move.
- o **Set New Challenges:** Periodically introduce new challenges or activities to keep your routine fresh and exciting.

By setting up a robust support system, utilizing tools and apps for tracking and reminders, and regularly revisiting and adjusting your goals, you can maintain your motivation and accountability throughout your weight loss journey.

Setting and Achieving Realistic, Measurable Goals

Setting realistic and achievable goals is crucial for successful weight loss and overall wellness. Here's how to do it effectively:

1. SMART Goals:

Specific: Clearly define your goal.
- o *Example:* "Lose 10 pounds."

Measurable: Track your progress.
- o *Example:* "Lose 1 pound per week."

Achievable: Ensure it's attainable.
- o *Example:* "Incorporate three 30-minute workouts per week."

Relevant: Make it meaningful to you.

o *Example:* "Improve my fitness to play with my kids more easily."

Time-bound: Set a deadline.

o *Example:* "Achieve this in 10 weeks."

2. Breaking Down Large Goals:

Chunk It: Divide big goals into smaller, actionable steps.

o *Example:* Instead of "Get fit," start with "Walk 10,000 steps daily."

Weekly Targets: Set weekly milestones.

o *Example:* "This week, replace sugary drinks with water."

3. Celebrating Small Victories:

Acknowledge Progress: Recognize and reward yourself for small achievements.

o *Example:* Treat yourself to a new book or a relaxing bath.

Stay Motivated: Celebrating small wins keeps you encouraged.

o *Example:* Share your success with friends or a support group.

By setting SMART goals, breaking them down into manageable steps, and celebrating small victories, you can stay motivated and steadily progress towards your weight loss and wellness objectives.

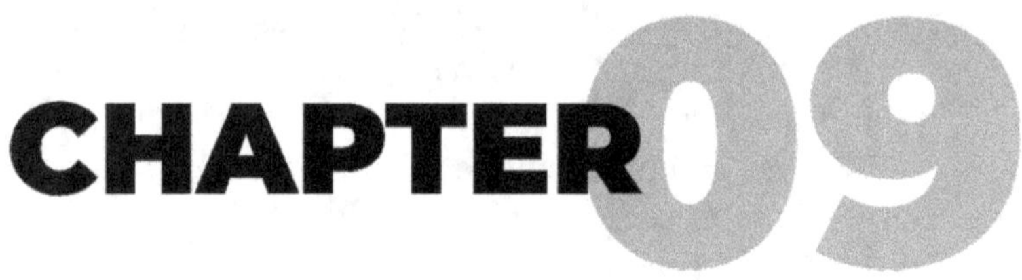

CHAPTER 09

MAINTAINING YOUR SUCCESS: STRATEGIES FOR LONG-TERM WELLNESS

As an experienced somatic coach, sustaining your wellness achievements requires a commitment to sustainable practices and lifestyle adjustments. Here's how to ensure continued success beyond the weight loss phase.

Building a Sustainable Somatic Practice

Integrating Somatic Exercises into Daily Routines

1. Daily Integration:

Micro-Sessions: Incorporate short sessions of somatic exercises throughout your day.
- *Example:* Start your morning with a 10-minute stretch routine, take breaks during work for gentle movements, and end the day with relaxation exercises.

Habit Stacking: Pair somatic exercises with daily habits.

- o *Example:* Perform neck rolls while waiting for your coffee to brew or practice deep breathing during your commute.

2. Consistency is Key:

Regular Schedule: Set aside specific times for your somatic practice.

- o *Example:* Dedicate 30 minutes every morning or evening for focused somatic exercise.

Routine Adherence: Treat your exercise time as a non-negotiable part of your day.

Variety and Moderation in Somatic Practices

1. Preventing Burnout:

Mix It Up: Keep your routine fresh by varying exercises.

- o *Example:* Alternate between yoga, Tai Chi, and Feldenkrais Method to target different muscle groups and keep things interesting.

Moderation: Balance intense workouts with gentle sessions.

- o *Example:* Follow a high-intensity session with a day of restorative movements.

2. Enjoyment and Interest:

Find What You Love: Engage in somatic practices that you enjoy and look forward to.

- o *Example:* If you love nature, incorporate outdoor sessions like mindful walking or Tai Chi in the park.
- **Set Challenges:** Periodically set new challenges or goals to maintain motivation.
  - o *Example:* Aim to master a new yoga pose or increase the duration of your meditation.

Continued Education and Adaptation

1. Lifelong Learning:

Stay Informed: Keep learning about new somatic techniques and practices.
- o *Example:* Attend workshops, read books, and follow expert blogs.

Seek Guidance: Work with a coach or join classes to refine your techniques and stay inspired.

2. Adaptation to Changing Needs:

Evolve Practices: Adapt your somatic exercises as your health and wellness needs change.
- o *Example:* Incorporate more strength-building exercises as you age or focus on flexibility if you develop stiffness.

Listen to Your Body: Regularly assess how your body feels and adjust your routine accordingly.
- o *Example:* If you notice new aches or stress, modify your practice to address these areas.

Navigating Life Transitions and Maintaining Weight Loss

Life transitions can present challenges to maintaining weight loss and wellness goals. Adapting to changes in lifestyle, environment, and circumstances requires strategic planning and a flexible mindset. Here are some strategies to help you stay on track.

Anticipating and Planning for Potential Disruptions

1. Travel:

> **Plan Ahead:** Research healthy food options and exercise facilities at your destination.
> - *Example:* Pack healthy snacks and find local gyms or walking routes.
>
> **Portable Workouts:** Bring exercise bands or use bodyweight exercises that can be done anywhere.
> - *Example:* Plan a 20-minute hotel room workout with squats, push-ups, and resistance band exercises.

2. Holidays:

> **Mindful Eating:** Practice portion control and savor holiday treats mindfully.
> - *Example:* Fill half your plate with vegetables before adding other foods.
>
> **Stay Active:** Incorporate physical activity into holiday traditions.
> - *Example:* Go for a family walk or play an active game after meals.

3. Workplace Challenges:

Healthy Choices: Pack balanced meals and snacks to avoid unhealthy cafeteria options.
- o *Example:* Prepare salads, whole-grain wraps, and fruit for your workday.

Active Breaks: Take short breaks to stretch or walk during the workday.
- o *Example:* Set a timer to remind you to stand and move every hour.

Flexible and Adaptable Mindset Towards Diet and Exercise

1. Embrace Flexibility:

Adjust Routines: Be open to modifying your diet and exercise routines as needed.
- o *Example:* If you miss a morning workout, do a shorter session in the evening.

Prioritize Balance: Allow yourself occasional indulgences without guilt.
- o *Example:* Enjoy a piece of cake at a celebration but balance it with a nutritious meal later.

2. Stay Positive:

Adapt Mindset: View challenges as opportunities to learn and grow.
- o *Example:* If you overeat at a party, use it as a learning experience to plan better next time.

Self-Compassion: Be kind to yourself and recognize that perfection is not the goal.
- o *Example:* Acknowledge your efforts and progress, even if there are setbacks.

Maintaining a Support Network for Motivation and Accountability

1. Build a Support Network:

Connect with Others: Share your goals with friends, family, or a support group.
- *Example:* Join a local or online weight loss support group for encouragement.

Accountability Partners: Find a workout buddy or a friend to share your journey.
- *Example:* Schedule regular check-ins with your accountability partner to stay on track.

Community and Support Systems

Finding or Creating Communities of Like-Minded Individuals

1. Local Groups:

Join Clubs: Look for local clubs focused on fitness, wellness, or nutrition.
- *Example:* Join a hiking club or a cooking class that emphasizes healthy eating.

Community Events: Participate in local wellness events or fitness challenges.
- *Example:* Sign up for charity walks or runs.

2. Online Communities:

Virtual Support: Join online forums, social media groups, or fitness apps to connect with others.
- *Example:* Participate in online challenges and share your progress with the group.

Resource Sharing: Use online platforms to exchange tips, recipes, and workout ideas.
- o *Example:* Follow fitness influencers or wellness coaches who inspire you.

The Benefits of Mentorship, Coaching, and Group Activities

1. Mentorship and Coaching:

Seek Guidance: Find a mentor or coach to provide personalized advice and support.
- o *Example:* Hire a personal trainer or nutritionist to help tailor your plan.

Ongoing Support: Regular sessions with a coach can help you stay focused and motivated.
- o *Example:* Schedule weekly check-ins to discuss progress and adjust goals.

2. Group Exercises and Activities:

Join Classes: Participate in group fitness classes or activities.
- o *Example:* Enroll in yoga, Zumba, or spinning classes at your local gym.

Social Interaction: Group settings provide a sense of community and accountability.
- o *Example:* Make friends in your fitness class to create a supportive environment.

Online and Virtual Platforms as Resources

1. Online Resources:

Virtual Workouts: Access a variety of workout videos and programs online.

- o *Example:* Use platforms like YouTube or fitness apps to find guided workouts.

Educational Content: Learn from webinars, online courses, and health blogs.

- o *Example:* Follow nutrition blogs or attend virtual workshops on wellness topics.

2. Inspiration and Support:

Follow Influencers: Get inspired by following fitness and wellness influencers.

- o *Example:* Subscribe to social media accounts that offer motivational content and tips.

Join Challenges: Participate in virtual fitness or wellness challenges.

- o *Example:* Join a 30-day fitness challenge hosted by an online community.

CHAPTER 10

HOLISTIC WELLNESS: BEYOND WEIGHT LOSS

Expanding the concept of wellness to encompass mental, emotional, and spiritual health alongside physical fitness provides a more comprehensive approach to well-being. This chapter delves into the broader benefits of adopting a holistic lifestyle and how it can significantly enhance your quality of life.

The Broader Benefits of a Holistic Lifestyle for Health and Well-being

Increased Energy and Vitality

1. Balanced Diet:

> **Nutrient-Dense Foods:** Consuming a diet rich in fruits, vegetables, lean proteins, and whole grains ensures your body receives essential vitamins and minerals.
>
> > o *Example:* Incorporating a variety of colorful vegetables and fruits into your meals can boost energy levels and improve overall health.

Steady Energy: Eating balanced meals at regular intervals helps maintain steady blood sugar levels, preventing energy crashes.

- o *Example:* A balanced breakfast with protein, healthy fats, and complex carbohydrates sets a positive tone for the day.

2. Regular Exercise:

Physical Activity: Engaging in regular exercise, including somatic practices, enhances cardiovascular health, muscle strength, and endurance.

- o *Example:* A mix of aerobic exercises, strength training, and flexibility workouts ensures a well-rounded fitness routine.

Vitality Boost: Regular physical activity increases the production of endorphins, which boosts energy and mood.

- o *Example:* Incorporating morning stretches or a brisk walk can invigorate your day and elevate your energy levels.

Improved Mental Health and Reduced Stress

1. Mindfulness and Meditation:

Stress Reduction: Practicing mindfulness and meditation helps lower cortisol levels, reduce stress, and promote relaxation.

- o *Example:* Daily meditation sessions, even for just 10 minutes, can significantly reduce stress and anxiety.

Mental Clarity: These practices enhance focus, attention, and cognitive function, improving overall mental health.

o *Example:* Mindfulness exercises like deep breathing or body scanning can be integrated into your daily routine for mental clarity.

2. Emotional Well-being:

Self-Awareness: Mindfulness practices increase self-awareness, helping you recognize and manage emotions more effectively.
o *Example:* Journaling your thoughts and feelings can help you process emotions and develop a deeper understanding of yourself.

Resilience: Developing emotional resilience through mindfulness enables better-coping mechanisms in stressful situations.
o *Example:* Engaging in activities that promote emotional well-being, such as creative arts or spending time in nature, can enhance resilience.

Enhanced Self-Esteem and Body Image

1. Consistent Somatic Practice:

Body Connection: Regular somatic exercises deepen your connection with your body, fostering a positive body image.
o *Example:* Practices like yoga or Tai Chi enhance body awareness and appreciation, leading to a healthier self-image.

Self-Esteem: Achieving fitness goals through somatic practices boosts confidence and self-esteem.
o *Example:* Celebrating small victories in your fitness journey, such as mastering a new pose, can reinforce positive self-esteem.

2. Holistic Self-Care:

Overall Wellness: Incorporating holistic self-care routines, such as adequate sleep, hydration, and relaxation techniques, supports comprehensive well-being.

- *Example:* Establishing a bedtime routine that includes winding down activities like reading or a warm bath promotes better sleep and overall wellness.

Balanced Lifestyle: Maintaining a balanced lifestyle that addresses physical, mental, emotional, and spiritual needs leads to sustained health and happiness.

- *Example:* Regularly engaging in activities that nourish your mind, body, and spirit, like hobbies or social connections, contributes to holistic wellness.

By embracing a holistic approach to wellness, you can achieve a state of well -being that transcends mere physical appearance. This comprehensive lifestyle enhances your energy, mental health, emotional resilience, and self -esteem.

Integrating Somatic Practices into Daily Life for Overall Wellness

Incorporating somatic exercises and mindfulness into daily routines can significantly enhance overall well-being. Here are practical tips and strategies to help you integrate these practices into your everyday life, promoting a holistic sense of wellness.

Practical Ways to Integrate Mindfulness and Movement into Work Life and Leisure

1. Work Life:

> **Mindful Breaks:** Schedule short breaks throughout your workday to practice mindfulness or somatic exercises.
> - *Example:* Set a timer to remind you to take a 5-minute break every hour. During this time, practice deep breathing or gentle stretches at your desk.
>
> **Desk Exercises:** Incorporate simple exercises that can be done while seated or standing.
> - *Example:* Perform seated cat-cow stretches, shoulder rolls, or standing leg stretches to relieve tension and stay active.

2. Leisure:

> **Active Leisure Activities:** Choose leisure activities that involve movement and mindfulness.
> - *Example:* Engage in hobbies like gardening, hiking, or dancing, which combine physical activity with relaxation.
>
> **Mindful Moments:** Incorporate mindfulness into everyday tasks.
> - *Example:* Practice mindful eating by savoring each bite, or engage in mindful walking by paying attention to your surroundings and breath.

Creating Routines and Habits that Support Physical, Mental, and Emotional Health

1. Morning Routine:

Start Your Day with Movement: Begin your morning with a short somatic exercise session.

- *Example:* Spend 10 minutes doing yoga or Tai Chi to wake up your body and mind.

Set Intentions: Use mindfulness to set positive intentions for the day.

- *Example:* Spend a few minutes meditating on your goals and visualizing a successful day.

2. Evening Routine:

Wind Down with Relaxation: Incorporate calming somatic practices into your evening routine.

- *Example:* Practice gentle stretches or deep breathing exercises before bed to promote relaxation and better sleep.

Reflect on Your Day: Use mindfulness to review your day and release any lingering stress.

- *Example:* Spend a few minutes journaling about your experiences and expressing gratitude.

Adjusting Lifestyle Choices to Reflect Holistic Wellness Priorities

1. Balanced Diet:

Mindful Eating: Make conscious food choices that nourish your body and mind.

- *Example:* Plan balanced meals with a variety of nutrients and practice mindful eating to enjoy each meal fully.

Healthy Snacks: Keep healthy snacks readily available to support your wellness goals.

- *Example:* Stock up on fruits, nuts, and yogurt for easy access to nutritious options.

2. Social Connections:

Supportive Relationships: Cultivate relationships that support your holistic wellness journey.
- o *Example:* Spend time with friends and family who encourage healthy habits and provide emotional support.

Community Involvement: Engage with communities that share your wellness values.
- o *Example:* Join local or online groups focused on holistic health, mindfulness, or fitness.

Life after Achieving Your Weight Loss Goals: What's Next?

Achieving your weight loss goals is a significant milestone, but it's essential to continue setting new goals and exploring further avenues for growth and self-improvement.

Exploring New Hobbies and Interests that Align with a Holistic Lifestyle

1. Discovering New Passions:

Try New Activities: Explore hobbies that support your holistic wellness.
- o *Example:* Take up activities like painting, cooking healthy meals, or learning a musical instrument to keep your mind and body engaged.

Join Classes: Enroll in classes that interest you and promote personal growth.
- o *Example:* Attend workshops on mindfulness, nutrition, or creative arts to expand your skills and knowledge.

Setting Personal Development Goals Beyond Physical Health

1. Learning Objectives:

Pursue Education: Set goals to learn new skills or advance your knowledge in areas of interest.
- *Example:* Enroll in online courses, read books, or attend seminars related to your passions.

Career Development: Focus on professional growth and career objectives.
- *Example:* Seek opportunities for professional development, such as certifications or networking events.

2. Personal Growth:

Mindfulness Practices: Continue to deepen your mindfulness practices.
- *Example:* Incorporate meditation, journaling, or yoga into your daily routine to foster ongoing personal growth.

Self-Reflection: Regularly assess your goals and progress.
- *Example:* Set aside time for self-reflection to evaluate your achievements and set new intentions.

Maintaining Momentum in Personal Wellness

1. Continuous Exploration:

Stay Curious: Keep exploring new wellness practices and approaches.

- o *Example:* Experiment with different types of exercises, diets, and mindfulness techniques to find what works best for you.

Adapt to Changes: Be flexible and adapt your routines to fit changing circumstances.

- o *Example:* Adjust your exercise and wellness practices as your lifestyle, needs, and interests evolve.

2. Accountability and Support:

Seek Support: Maintain connections with your support network.

- o *Example:* Continue attending support groups, working with a coach, or engaging with wellness communities.

Track Progress: Use tools and apps to monitor your ongoing wellness journey.

- o *Example:* Keep a journal or use fitness apps to track your progress, set new goals, and stay motivated.

By integrating somatic practices into your daily life, setting new goals, and continuously exploring ways to improve, you can sustain your wellness achievements and enhance your overall quality of life.

CHAPTER 11

APPENDICES AND RESOURCES

This chapter provides supplemental materials to support your journey into somatic exercise and holistic wellness. Here, you will find detailed guides, meal plans, and resources to help you further explore and apply these principles in your daily life.

Detailed Guide to Somatic Exercises and Routines

Step-by-Step Guides for Core Somatic Movements

1. **Pelvic Tilts:**
   - **Description:** Lie on your back with your knees bent and feet flat on the floor. Gently tilt your pelvis towards your belly button, then back towards the floor.
   - **Benefits:** Releases lower back tension and strengthens the core.
   - **Visual Aid:** Include diagrams or photos of each step.

2. **Cat-Cow Stretch:**
   - **Description:** On hands and knees, alternate between arching your back (Cow) and rounding it (Cat).
   - **Benefits:** Enhances spinal flexibility and relieves tension.
   - **Visual Aid:** Step-by-step illustrations.
3. **Shoulder Rolls:**
   - **Description:** Sit or stand comfortably. Slowly roll your shoulders up, back, down, and forward in a circular motion.
   - **Benefits:** Relieves shoulder tension and improves mobility.
   - **Visual Aid:** Demonstrative images.

Video Tutorials and Demonstrations

1. **Access to Tutorials:**
   - **Links to Videos:** Provide URLs to video tutorials for each core somatic exercise.
   - **Description:** Brief descriptions of what each video covers.
2. **Demonstration Platforms:**
   - **YouTube Channels:** Recommend reliable channels that focus on somatic exercises.
   - **App Integration:** Suggest apps with instructional videos and guided routines.

Variations of Exercises for Different Skill Levels

1. **Beginner Variations:**

- o **Modification Tips:** Offer simpler versions of exercises for those new to somatic practice.
  - o **Example:** Gentle pelvic tilts instead of full hip bridges.
2. **Intermediate Variations:**
   - o **Enhanced Movements:** Introduce slightly more challenging variations.
   - o **Example:** Adding resistance bands to shoulder rolls.
3. **Advanced Variations:**
   - o **Intensified Exercises:** Provide advanced modifications for experienced practitioners.
   - o **Example:** Combining Cat-Cow stretch with leg lifts for added core engagement.

Comprehensive Meal Plans and Recipes

Weekly Meal Plans Incorporating Mindful Eating

1. **Sample Weekly Plan:**
   - o **Breakfast:** Smoothies, overnight oats, whole-grain toast with avocado.
   - o **Lunch:** Quinoa salad, vegetable wraps, grilled chicken with mixed greens.
   - o **Dinner:** Baked salmon with roasted vegetables, stir-fried tofu with brown rice.
   - o **Snacks:** Nuts, fruits, yoghurt.
2. **Mindful Eating Tips:**
   - o **Portion Control:** Encourage smaller, more frequent meals.
   - o **Mindful Chewing:** Emphasize the importance of chewing slowly and savoring each bite.

Recipes Focused on Whole Foods

1. **Breakfast Recipes:**
    - o **Example:** Greek yogurt with honey, nuts, and berries.
    - o **Instructions:** Detailed steps and nutritional information.
2. **Lunch Recipes:**
    - o **Example:** Quinoa and black bean salad.
    - o **Instructions:** Ingredients, preparation steps, and tips for variations.
3. **Dinner Recipes:**
    - o **Example:** Grilled chicken with roasted sweet potatoes and steamed broccoli.
    - o **Instructions:** Easy-to-follow steps with cooking tips.
4. **Snack Recipes:**
    - o **Example:** Hummus with vegetable sticks.
    - o **Instructions:** Simple, quick recipes for healthy snacking.

Tips for Meal Prep and Cooking Techniques

1. **Meal Prep Strategies:**
    - o **Batch Cooking:** Cook large quantities and store portions for the week.
    - o **Organization:** Use labeled containers to keep meals organized.
2. **Cooking Techniques:**
    - o **Healthy Methods:** Focus on baking, steaming, and grilling instead of frying.
    - o **Flavor Enhancements:** Use herbs and spices to enhance flavor without added fats or sugars.

CONCLUSION

As we conclude this comprehensive guide on somatic exercises, mindful eating, and holistic wellness, it is essential to acknowledge the profound impact these practices can have on your overall well-being. This journey is not just about losing weight but about embracing a lifestyle that fosters physical, mental, and emotional health.

The integration of somatic exercises into your daily routine enhances body awareness, reduces stress, and improves physical fitness. By focusing on mindful movements and connecting with your body, you can develop a deeper understanding of its needs and capabilities. This heightened awareness enables you to move more efficiently, reduce the risk of injury, and experience greater physical comfort and vitality.

Mindful eating complements these physical practices by encouraging a balanced and thoughtful approach to nutrition. By paying attention to hunger and fullness cues, you can make healthier food choices, avoid overeating, and foster a positive relationship with food. Incorporating whole foods into your diet supports sustained energy levels, better digestion, and overall improved health.

Holistic wellness extends beyond physical practices to include mental and emotional well-being. Mindfulness and meditation are powerful tools for managing stress, enhancing mental clarity, and fostering emotional resilience. These practices help you stay present, reduce anxiety, and cultivate a sense of inner peace.

Setting realistic and measurable goals is crucial for maintaining motivation and tracking progress. Breaking down larger objectives into smaller, manageable steps ensures continuous improvement and sustained success. Celebrate your achievements along the way to reinforce positive behaviors and maintain momentum.

Building a support system is equally important. Engage with communities and seek guidance from mentors or coaches to stay motivated and accountable. Sharing your journey with others provides encouragement and inspiration.

In summary, integrating somatic exercises, mindful eating, and holistic wellness practices into your daily life leads to comprehensive health improvements. Embrace this journey with curiosity and self-compassion, recognizing it as an opportunity for profound personal growth and enhanced quality of life. Stay committed to your goals, adapt to changes, and continue exploring new avenues for self-improvement. Your path to holistic wellness is a lifelong adventure, rich with benefits for your body, mind, and spirit.